BLOOD TYPE

B

DIET COOKBOOK

A Beginner's Guide to Personalized
Eating for Health With Wholesome
Recipes and Tips

Jade E.Corry

TABLE OF CONTENTS

INTRODUCTION

Welcome to the culinary journey that promises to transform the way you think about food and its profound impact on your well-being. In the pages of this cookbook, I invite you to explore the world of the Blood Type B diet—a dietary approach grounded in personalized nutrition and designed to unlock the secrets of your unique genetic blueprint.

At its core, the Blood Type B diet reflects the belief that our blood type shapes not only our physiology but also our dietary requirements. For those with Blood Type B, this journey is a revelation of a holistic approach to health, one that considers not just what we eat but also how our bodies interact with the foods we choose.

Our mission is simple: to empower you with the knowledge, tools, and delectable recipes that will enable you to thrive on the Blood Type B diet. From revitalizing breakfasts to satisfying dinners and tempting desserts, each recipe is thoughtfully crafted to align with the principles of this distinctive dietary philosophy.

As you turn the pages, you'll discover the origins, core principles, and science behind the Blood Type B diet, all presented in a unique and engaging way. Our aim is to demystify the diet, making it accessible and enjoyable for individuals seeking a path to wellness tailored to their blood type.

Prepare to embark on a culinary adventure that not only tantalizes your taste buds but also nurtures your health. Embrace the Blood Type B diet, and let these recipes become your passport to a healthier, more vibrant you. Whether you're a seasoned follower of the diet or a newcomer intrigued by its potential, this cookbook is your guide to personalized wellness through the art of nourishing cuisine.

Understanding the Blood Type B Diet

The Blood Type B diet is a distinctive and personalized dietary approach that has gained attention for its potential to promote health and well-being based on an individual's blood type. This dietary philosophy is rooted in the belief that our blood type influences our body's ability to digest and utilize certain foods, and as a result, can impact our overall health.

In this exploration, we will delve into the origins, core principles, and design of the Blood Type B diet, shedding light on its unique nature.

The Origins and Theory

The concept of the Blood Type B diet is grounded in the broader framework of the Blood Type Diet, developed by Dr. Peter D'Adamo in the late 1990s. Dr. D'Adamo's theory posits that one's blood type, specifically Types A, B, AB, and O, determines how our bodies interact with foods, impacting everything from digestion to disease susceptibility.

The Blood Type B diet, in particular, caters to individuals with Blood Type B, offering them a dietary blueprint tailored to their unique genetic makeup.

CHAPTER 1: BLOOD TYPE B DIET BASICS

In this chapter,You will get to know unique traits and characteristics associated with individuals who have Blood Type B. Explore how these traits may influence their dietary needs and health.

Blood Type B Traits and Characteristics

Blood Type B individuals possess a distinct genetic makeup that sets them apart in terms of traits, characteristics, and potential dietary needs. Understanding these unique features is crucial for tailoring a diet that optimizes their health and well-being.

Flexibility and Adaptability:
- **Characteristic**: Blood Type B individuals are often described as having a flexible digestive system. This adaptability enables them to process a wide range of foods more easily than some other blood types.

- **Dietary Influence**: Their digestive resilience allows for a diverse diet that includes various food groups. However, it's essential to focus on foods that align with their blood type to maintain digestive harmony.

Resilient Immune System:

- **Characteristic**: Blood Type B individuals are believed to have a resilient immune system, offering efficient protection against certain illnesses.
- **Dietary Influence**: While their immune resilience is an advantage, maintaining overall health remains vital. A diet rich in immune-boosting nutrients can complement their inherent strength.

Sensitivity to Stress:

- **Characteristic**: Blood Type B individuals may exhibit increased sensitivity to stressors, making stress management a critical aspect of their overall health.

- **Dietary Influence**: A diet that includes stress-reducing foods like leafy greens, lean meats, and certain herbs can help mitigate the impact of stress on their well-being.

Potential Vulnerabilities:

- **Characteristic**: Blood Type B individuals may be more prone to certain health challenges, including autoimmune disorders and inflammation-related conditions.
- **Dietary Influence**: Their dietary choices can play a pivotal role in managing these vulnerabilities. Avoiding foods that may exacerbate inflammation and incorporating anti-inflammatory options can be beneficial.

Exercise Preferences:

- **Characteristic**: Blood Type B individuals often exhibit preferences for activities that promote balance and flexibility, such as yoga and tai chi.
- **Dietary Influence**: Their diet can complement these preferences by providing the energy and nutrients needed for these activities.

Potential Allergies and Intolerances:
- **Characteristic**: Some Blood Type B individuals may be susceptible to specific food allergies and intolerances.
- **Dietary Influence**: Identifying and avoiding allergenic or problematic foods is crucial for maintaining digestive comfort and overall health.

Personalizing Your Diet

Key Elements of Personalization:

- **Blood Type-Based Personalization:** One intriguing approach to personalization is the Blood Type Diet, which suggests that your blood type influences how your body interacts with certain foods. For instance, individuals with blood type A may find that a plant-based diet aligns well with their physiology, while those with blood type O might thrive on a diet that includes more animal products.
- **Metabolic Typing:** Metabolic typing takes into account your metabolic rate and how your body processes macronutrients.

It classifies individuals as fast oxidizers (better with fats and proteins) or slow oxidizers (who may do better with carbohydrates). This approach guides dietary choices to match your metabolic type.

- **Food Sensitivity Testing:**

Food sensitivity tests can identify specific foods or food groups that may trigger adverse reactions in your body. Avoiding these foods can alleviate symptoms like digestive issues, headaches, or skin problems.

- **Nutrient Needs:**

Personalization considers your individual nutrient requirements, ensuring that you meet your daily recommended intake of essential vitamins and minerals. Some individuals may require specific supplements to fill nutritional gaps.

Benefits of a Personalized Diet:

- **Enhanced Nutrient Absorption:**

A personalized diet is tailored to your body's ability to absorb and utilize nutrients, ensuring that you receive the maximum benefit from the foods you consume.

- **Improved Digestion**:
Foods that align with your body's digestive capabilities reduce the risk of digestive discomfort and promote a healthy gut.

- **Weight Management**:
Personalization can be particularly effective for weight management, as it aligns dietary choices with your metabolic rate and energy needs.

- **Optimized Athletic Performance:**
Athletes can benefit from a personalized diet that fuels their training, improves recovery, and supports muscle growth.

- **Disease Management:**
Personalized diets can be instrumental in managing chronic conditions like diabetes, celiac disease, or food allergies. They help avoid trigger foods and provide essential nutrients.

The Science of Blood Type and Diet

One of the foundational theories supporting the Blood Type Diet suggests that blood types, including Type B, may have evolved in response to dietary and environmental factors. For instance, individuals with blood Type B are believed to have ancestral roots in regions where agriculture and the domestication of animals were prevalent. This historical perspective suggests that the digestive capabilities of Type B individuals adapted to accommodate a more diverse diet that included both plant-based and animal-based foods.

Some studies have explored the relationship between blood type and the immune system. It's theorized that different blood types may influence the body's response to infections and diseases. For example, research suggests that individuals with blood Type B may have different immune responses to certain pathogens and infections compared to those with other blood types.

While the scientific foundation of the Blood Type B diet is intriguing, it's important to acknowledge that the concept is met with varying degrees of acceptance in the scientific community. Critics argue that more robust, well-controlled studies are needed to definitively establish the links between blood type, dietary lectins, and health outcomes. The diet's personalized approach, however, has found proponents who report positive health outcomes.

The Role of Lectins

The Blood Type B diet, a key element of the broader Blood Type Diet framework, is underpinned by a unique set of theories and scientific concepts. One of the central ideas is the role of lectins in influencing how different blood types react to specific foods. Beyond this, various theories surrounding genetics, digestion, and health outcomes contribute to the foundation of the diet. Let's explore these theories and the role of lectins in greater detail.

At the core of the Blood Type Diet, the theory of lectins takes center stage. Lectins are proteins found in a wide range of foods, including grains, legumes, and certain vegetables. The fundamental premise of this theory is that lectins can interact with the antigens present on the surface of red blood cells. Depending on an individual's blood type, these interactions can have varying effects on health.

For individuals with Blood Type B, the theory suggests that their blood type antigens are less reactive to certain lectins commonly found in foods like meats, fish, and dairy. This reduced reactivity is believed to make these individuals more tolerant of these food sources, enabling better digestion and overall health. Conversely, foods that contain lectins that are less compatible with Type B blood are advised to be minimized or avoided.

The Blood Type Diet asserts that blood types may be linked to evolutionary and genetic factors. For instance, it posits that Type B individuals have a genetic heritage associated with regions where agriculture and the domestication of animals were prominent.

Over time, their digestive systems adapted to process a broader spectrum of foods, both plant-based and animal-based, as their ancestors transitioned to agrarian societies. This adaptation is believed to have influenced the dietary needs and tolerances of individuals with Blood Type B.

The Role of Fucose:
Recent research has explored the role of the Fucose antigen, which is associated with Blood Type B. It's theorized that Fucose can interact with certain strains of gut bacteria, influencing the composition of the gut microbiome. This interplay between Fucose and gut bacteria is believed to have implications for immune function and overall health. While this area of research is still emerging, it adds another layer to the intricate relationship between blood type and dietary requirements.

Blood Type and Digestion
The idea that blood type may influence how our bodies digest food and absorb nutrients is a central tenet of the Blood Type Diet, which suggests that dietary choices should be tailored to an individual's specific blood type.

While this concept is not universally accepted within the scientific community, it offers a unique perspective on the interplay between genetics, physiology, and nutrition. Let's explore how blood type affects digestion and nutrient absorption and delve into the scientific theories that underlie these connections.

Blood type is determined by the presence or absence of specific antigens on the surface of red blood cells. There are four main blood types: A, B, AB, and O, each with distinct antigens. These blood type antigens, especially the ABO and Rh systems, play a critical role in blood transfusions and organ transplantation compatibility. The Blood Type Diet posits that these antigens also influence how our bodies interact with food.

The Blood Type Diet also considers the role of digestive enzymes in breaking down and processing food. It suggests that individuals with Type B blood possess specific enzymes well-suited for the digestion of animal proteins. This theory is predicated on the idea that their digestive system is better equipped to handle these proteins efficiently.

Additionally, the diet proposes that individuals with Type B blood have an enhanced capacity for absorbing particular nutrients, such as calcium and magnesium, from dairy products, further influencing their dietary requirements.

The Blood Type Diet posits that individuals with blood Type B have specific digestive enzymes that are well-suited for the foods recommended in their diet. For instance, Type B individuals are believed to produce adequate stomach acid, which aids in the digestion of animal proteins.

CHAPTER 2: FOODS FOR BLOOD TYPE B

Blood Type B Food List

The Blood Type B diet is designed to align with the unique traits and characteristics of individuals with Blood Type B. While it's essential to consult with a healthcare professional or registered dietitian before making significant dietary changes, here's a comprehensive list of foods that are generally recommended for those with Blood Type B:

Foods to Embrace for Blood Type B

1.Proteins

- **Lean Meats**: Choose lean cuts of beef, lamb, rabbit, venison, and game meats. These are rich in essential nutrients and align well with the Blood Type B digestive system.

- **Poultry**: Opt for turkey, duck, and quail. These poultry options are generally well-tolerated by Blood Type B individuals.

- **Fish**: Include salmon, halibut, mackerel, mahi-mahi, trout, and sardines in your diet. They provide quality protein and healthy fats.

- **Dairy**: Consume yogurt, kefir, goat's milk, and certain cheeses like feta and mozzarella. These dairy products are typically easier on digestion.

2.Vegetables

- **Green Leafy Vegetables**: Incorporate kale, spinach, and lettuce into your meals. They are excellent sources of vitamins and minerals.

- **Cruciferous Vegetables**: Include broccoli and Brussels sprouts in your diet, as they offer numerous health benefits.

- **Colorful Vegetables**: Carrots, beets, sweet potatoes, and onions provide variety and nutrients to your meals.

3.Fruits

- **Berries**: Blueberries, blackberries, cranberries, and other berries are rich in antioxidants and vitamins.

- **Tropical Fruits**: Enjoy papaya, plums, pineapple, grapes, and cherries for a sweet and nutritious treat.

4.Grains and Starches
- **Oat Bran**: Oat bran is an excellent source of fiber and can be a healthy addition to your diet.

Moderate Amounts of Rice: While rice is generally fine, consume it in moderation.

- **Whole Grains**: Opt for whole grains like millet, quinoa, buckwheat, and spelt, which offer fiber and nutrients.

5.Legumes
- **Lentils**: Lentils are a good source of plant-based protein and fiber.
- **Green Peas and Black-Eyed Peas**: These legumes can be included in your diet in moderation.

6.Nuts and Seeds

- **Almonds and Walnuts**: Almonds and walnuts provide healthy fats and are excellent for snacking.

- **Flaxseeds and Sunflower Seeds**: These seeds offer nutritional value and can be sprinkled on salads or yogurt.

7.Oils

- **Olive Oil:** Olive oil is a healthy source of monounsaturated fats that can be used for cooking and as a salad dressing.

- **Flaxseed Oil:** Flaxseed oil is rich in omega-3 fatty acids, contributing to overall health.

- **Ghee (Clarified Butter):** In moderation, ghee can add flavor to your dishes.

8.Herbs and Spices:

- **Turmeric, Parsley, Dill, Ginger, and Red Pepper Flakes:** These herbs and spices can enhance the flavor of your meals while offering potential health benefits.

9.Beverages

- **Green Tea:** Green tea is known for its antioxidant properties and can be a healthy beverage choice.

- **Herbal Teas:** Options like chamomile can provide a soothing and caffeine-free alternative.

10.Sweeteners

- **Honey and Maple Syrup**: These natural sweeteners can be used in moderation to add a touch of sweetness to your recipes.

Foods to Avoid for Blood Type B

1.**Chicken**: Limit or avoid chicken, as it's believed to be less compatible with the Blood Type B digestive system.

2.**Corn**: Corn is considered less favorable for Blood Type B individuals due to its lectin content.

3.Lentils: While lentils can be included in moderation, some Blood Type B individuals may find them less digestible.

4.Peanuts: Peanuts and peanut products may not align well with the Blood Type B diet due to lectins.

5.Sesame Seeds: Sesame seeds and sesame oil are recommended to be limited or avoided.

6.Tomatoes: Some individuals with Blood Type B may have sensitivities to tomatoes.

The Healing Power of Blood Type B Foods

The Blood Type B-friendly foods, as recommended by the Blood Type Diet, encompass a diverse array of nutrient-rich options that can contribute to overall health and well-being. Let's delve into the nutritional profiles of these foods and their potential health benefits:

1.Lean Meats (Beef, Lamb, Rabbit, Venison):

- **Protein**: Lean meats are excellent sources of high-quality protein, vital for muscle development and tissue repair.

- **Iron**: They provide heme iron, which is easily absorbed and helps prevent anemia.

- **Zinc**: Zinc supports immune function and wound healing.

- **B Vitamins**: These meats contain essential B vitamins, including B12, necessary for energy metabolism and nerve health.

2.Poultry (Turkey, Duck, Quail):

- **Protein**: Poultry offers lean protein, crucial for maintaining muscle and overall health.

- **Selenium**: Selenium is essential for protecting cells from oxidative damage.

- B Vitamins: Turkey, for instance, is a source of B vitamins, including niacin, supporting cardiovascular health.

3.Fish (Salmon, Halibut, Mackerel, Mahi-mahi, Trout, Sardines):

- **Omega-3 Fatty Acids**: These fish are rich in omega-3s, which are linked to heart health, reduced inflammation, and improved cognitive function.

- **Protein**: Fish provides high-quality protein while being low in saturated fat.

- **Vitamins**: They contain essential vitamins, including vitamin D, which is important for bone health.

4.Dairy (Yogurt, Kefir, Goat's Milk, Feta, Mozzarella:

- **Calcium**: Dairy is a prime source of calcium, critical for strong bones and teeth.

- **Probiotics**: Yogurt and kefir are rich in probiotics, beneficial for gut health and digestion.

- **Protein**: Dairy products supply protein, contributing to muscle and tissue health.

- **Vitamins**: They provide vitamins like B12, essential for nerve function.

5.Fruits (Berries, Papaya, Plums, Pineapple, Grapes, Cherries):

- **Antioxidants**: Berries are packed with antioxidants that combat free radicals and reduce the risk of chronic diseases.

- **Fiber**: Fruits offer dietary fiber, promoting digestive health and aiding weight management.

- **Vitamins**: They contain an array of vitamins, including vitamin C, which boosts the immune system.

6. Vegetables (Green Leafy, Cruciferous, Colorful:

- **Fiber**: Vegetables are rich in fiber, promoting satiety and digestive regularity.

- **Phytonutrients**: They contain phytonutrients that have potential health benefits, such as sulforaphane in broccoli, known for its cancer-fighting properties.

- **Vitamins**: Vegetables provide essential vitamins like vitamin K and vitamin A, supporting bone and eye health.

7. Grains and Starches (Oat Bran, Rice, Millet, Quinoa, Buckwheat, Spelt:

- **Fiber**: Whole grains are excellent sources of dietary fiber, promoting digestive health.

- **Complex Carbohydrates**: They provide a steady source of energy and help maintain blood sugar levels.

- **B Vitamins**: Grains offer various B vitamins, contributing to metabolism and overall health.

8.Legumes (Lentils, Green Peas, Black-Eyed Peas):

- **Protein**: Legumes are plant-based protein sources, suitable for vegetarians.

- **Fiber**: They are high in dietary fiber, aiding digestion and promoting fullness.

- **Minerals**: Legumes supply essential minerals, including iron and folate.

9.Nuts and Seeds (Almonds, Walnuts, Flaxseeds, Sunflower Seeds):

- **Healthy Fats:** Nuts and seeds provide heart-healthy monounsaturated and polyunsaturated fats.

- **Protein**: They are sources of plant-based protein, contributing to muscle health.

- **Fiber**: Nuts and seeds contain dietary fiber, supporting digestive health.

10.Oils (Olive Oil, Flaxseed Oil, Ghee):

- **Healthy Fats**: These oils offer healthy fats, including monounsaturated and omega-3 fatty acids, benefiting heart and brain health.

- **Antioxidants**: Olive oil, in particular, is rich in antioxidants, reducing inflammation and oxidative stress.

11.Herbs and Spices (Turmeric, Parsley, Dill, Ginger, Red Pepper Flakes:

- **Anti-Inflammatory Properties**: Many herbs and spices possess anti-inflammatory properties, potentially reducing the risk of chronic diseases.

- **Antioxidants**: They contain antioxidants that protect cells from damage.

- **Digestive Benefits**: Some herbs and spices aid digestion and alleviate gastrointestinal discomfort.

12. Beverages (Green Tea, Herbal Teas):

- **Antioxidants**: Green tea and herbal teas are rich in antioxidants, promoting overall health and reducing the risk of chronic diseases.

- **Hydration**: Staying well-hydrated is essential for maintaining bodily functions and overall health.

13. Sweeteners (Honey and Maple Syrup):

- **Natural Sweeteners:** Honey and maple syrup are natural sweeteners that provide a touch of sweetness to dishes.

Meal Planning for Blood Type B

Creating balanced and satisfying meals that align with the Blood Type B diet can be both enjoyable and nutritious. Here's practical guidance to help you plan your meals:

1. **Protein Selection**:
   - Start with a lean protein source, such as beef, lamb, turkey, or fish.
   - Opt for smaller portion sizes to maintain balance in your meal.
   - Consider marinating proteins in olive oil, herbs, and spices for added flavor.

2. **Vegetable Variety:**
   - Build your meal around a foundation of vegetables. Include green leafy greens, cruciferous vegetables like broccoli, and colorful options such as carrots and beets.
   - Steam, roast, or sauté your vegetables to preserve their nutrients and flavors.
   - Experiment with different seasonings and herbs for a diverse taste.

3. **Whole Grains and Starches:**
   - Incorporate whole grains like quinoa or buckwheat, which are rich in fiber and nutrients.
   - Use starches like sweet potatoes or brown rice sparingly to maintain balance in your meal.
   - Create grain-based salads or side dishes with fresh herbs and lemon.

4. **Dairy or Dairy Alternatives**:
   - Include yogurt or kefir in your meal for a creamy and probiotic-rich side.
   - For dairy alternatives, choose goat's milk or dairy-free yogurt if preferred.
   - Use dairy products to create sauces or dressings for added flavor.

5. **Fruit Additions**:
   - Include a serving of fruits, such as berries, papaya, or plums, as a side or dessert.
   - Mix fruits into salads or enjoy them as a refreshing snack.
   - Avoid excessive consumption of high-sugar fruits to maintain balance.

6. **Nuts and Seeds:**
- Sprinkle chopped almonds or walnuts on salads or vegetables for added texture and healthy fats.
- Use flaxseeds or sunflower seeds as a garnish or in smoothies.
- Remember that nuts and seeds are calorie-dense, so use them in moderation.

7. **Healthy Cooking Oils**:
- Use olive oil for sautéing or drizzle it over vegetables for added flavor.
- Try flaxseed oil as a finishing touch on salads for a dose of omega-3 fatty acids.
- Consider using ghee as a butter alternative for cooking or baking.

8. **Herbs and Spices:**
- Season your meals with herbs and spices like turmeric, parsley, ginger, or red pepper flakes.
- Experiment with combinations to enhance the flavor profile of your dishes.
- Herbs and spices not only add taste but also offer potential health benefits.

9. **Beverages**:
- Choose green tea or herbal teas as beverages, which can complement your meal.
- Avoid excessive caffeine or sugary drinks to maintain the overall balance of your diet.
- Stay well-hydrated throughout the day by consuming ample water.

Portion Control:

Be mindful of portion sizes, as overeating can disrupt the balance of your meals.Consider using smaller plates to help with portion control. Listen to your body's hunger and fullness cues.

Sample Meal Plans

Here's a sample meal plan for a day that aligns with the Blood Type B diet. Keep in mind that this is just one example, and you can create a variety of meal plans based on your preferences and dietary needs.

Day 1: Sample Meal Plan for Blood Type B

Breakfast
- Greek yogurt with a handful of fresh berries (blueberries, blackberries, or strawberries).
- A sprinkle of crushed flaxseeds for added fiber and omega-3 fatty acids.
- Green tea or herbal tea.

Lunch
- Grilled turkey breast or turkey burger (seasoned with herbs and spices) served on a bed of leafy greens (kale and spinach).
- Sautéed broccoli and carrots in olive oil with a touch of ginger for added flavor.
- Quinoa salad with diced cucumbers, red bell peppers, and parsley, dressed with a simple lemon and olive oil vinaigrette.
- A glass of water with a squeeze of lemon.

Snack
- A small handful of almonds or walnuts for a quick and satisfying snack.
- Fresh papaya or a plum for a sweet and hydrating option.

Dinner

- Baked salmon with a sprinkle of red pepper flakes for a touch of heat.
- Roasted sweet potatoes seasoned with a dash of paprika.
- A side salad with mixed greens, feta cheese, and a simple olive oil and vinegar dressing.
- Herbal tea for a soothing end to the day.

Snack (if needed):

- A cup of herbal tea or a glass of water
- A small portion of yogurt or a handful of cherries for a light, evening snack.

CHAPTER 3:BREAKFAST DELIGHTS FOR BLOOD TYPE B

QUICK WEEKDAY BREAKFASTS

Turkey and Veggie Scramble

Ingredients
- 2 eggs
- 1/4 cup diced turkey
- 1/4 cup diced bell peppers
- 1/4 cup diced onions

Preparation
- In a non-stick skillet, sauté turkey and vegetables until cooked.
- Beat eggs and pour them over the cooked ingredients.
- Scramble until eggs are set.

Nutritional Value
- Calories: 250-300
- Protein: 20-25g
- Carbohydrates: 5-10g
- Fat: 15-20g

Cooking Time

* 10 minutes

Green Smoothie

Ingredients

* 1 cup spinach
* 1/2 banana
* 1/2 cup papaya
* 1/2 cup almond milk

Preparation

* Blend all ingredients until smooth.

Nutritional Value

* Calories: 150-200
* Protein: 3-5g
* Carbohydrates: 30-35g
* Dietary Fiber: 5-7g

Cooking Time

* 5 minutes

Millet Porridge

Ingredients

* 1/2 cup cooked millet
* 1/4 cup diced plums

- 1 tablespoon chopped walnuts

Preparation
- Warm cooked millet.
- Top with plums and walnuts.

Nutritional Value
- Calories: 300-350
- Protein: 7-10g
- Carbohydrates: 45-50g
- Dietary Fiber: 5-7g

Cooking Time
10 minutes

Greek Yogurt Parfait

Ingredients
- 1 cup Greek yogurt
- 1/2 cup mixed berries (e.g., blueberries, blackberries, and strawberries)
- 1 tablespoon crushed flaxseeds
- 1 teaspoon honey (optional)

Preparation
Layer ingredients in a glass.

Nutritional Value
- Calories: 350-400
- Protein: 20-25g
- Carbohydrates: 30-35g
- Dietary Fiber: 8-10g

- Sugars: 15-20g (from natural sugars in berries and yogurt)
- Fat: 15-20g
- Omega-3 Fatty Acids: 2-3g (from flaxseeds)

Cooking Time

- 5-10 minutes

Omelet with Smoked Salmon

Ingredients

- 2 eggs
- 1/4 cup diced smoked salmon
- 1/4 cup chopped dill

Preparation

- Whisk eggs, then pour them into a heated, non-stick skillet.
- Add smoked salmon and dill.
- Cook until set.

Nutritional Value

- Calories: 250-300
- Protein: 20-25g
- Carbohydrates: 2-5g
- Fat: 15-20g

Cooking Time

- 10 minutes

WEEKEND BRUNCH OPTIONS

Buckwheat Pancakes

Ingredients
- 1 cup buckwheat flour
- 1/2 teaspoon baking powder
- 1 egg
- 1 cup almond milk

Preparation
- Mix buckwheat flour and baking powder.
- In a separate bowl, beat the egg and combine it with almond milk.
- Stir the wet ingredients into the dry to make the pancake batter.
- Cook the pancakes on a hot griddle.

Nutritional Value
- Calories: 300-350
- Protein: 8-10g
- Carbohydrates: 45-50g
- Dietary Fiber: 6-8g
- Sugars: 2-5g
- Fat: 10-15g

Cooking Time
20 minutes.

Quinoa Breakfast Bowl

Ingredients

- 1/2 cup cooked quinoa
- 1/4 cup sautéed vegetables (e.g., zucchini, bell peppers, onions)
- 1 poached egg
- 1 teaspoon olive oil

Preparation

- Warm the cooked quinoa.
- Top with sautéed vegetables and a poached egg.
- Drizzle with olive oil.

Nutritional Value

- Calories: 300-350
- Protein: 10-15g
- Carbohydrates: 25-30g
- Dietary Fiber: 4-6g
- Fat: 15-20

Cooking Time

- 15 minutes

Vegetable Frittata

Ingredients

- 4 eggs
- 1 cup mixed vegetables (e.g., zucchini, bell peppers, onions)
- 1/2 teaspoon ground ginger
- 1/4 teaspoon red pepper flakes

Preparation

- In an oven-safe skillet, sauté vegetables with ginger and red pepper flakes.
- Beat eggs and pour them over the cooked vegetables.
- Transfer the skillet to the oven and bake until set.

Nutritional Value

- Calories: 300-350
- Protein: 12-15g
- Carbohydrates: 10-15g
- Dietary Fiber: 2-4g
- Fat: 15-20g

Cooking Time

- 20 minutes

Pineapple Coconut Smoothie

Ingredients

- 1 cup fresh pineapple
- 1/2 cup coconut milk
- 1 scoop protein powder

Preparation

- Blend all ingredients until smooth.

Nutritional Value

- Calories: 250-300
- Protein: 15-20g
- Carbohydrates: 20-25g
- Dietary Fiber: 2-4g

Cooking Time

- 5 minutes

Smoked Salmon Benedict

Ingredients

- 2 whole-grain English muffins
- 1/2 cup smoked salmon
- 2 poached eggs
- 1/4 cup Greek yogurt
- 1 tablespoon chopped dill

Preparation

- Toast English muffins.
- Top each half with smoked salmon, a poached egg, and a dollop of Greek yogurt.
- Sprinkle with dill.

Nutritional Value

- Calories: 350-400
- Protein: 25-30g
- Carbohydrates: 25-30g
- Dietary Fiber: 5-7g
- Fat: 15-20g

Cooking Time

- 15 minutes

Lentil Breakfast Bowl

Ingredients

- 1/2 cup cooked lentils
- 1/4 cup sautéed vegetables (e.g., zucchini, bell peppers, onions)
- 1 fried egg
- 1 tablespoon chopped parsley

Preparation

- Warm the cooked lentils.
- Top with sautéed vegetables and a fried egg.

- Sprinkle with chopped parsley.

Nutritional Value

- Calories: 350-400
- Protein: 15-20g
- Carbohydrates: 35-40g
- Dietary Fiber: 6-8g
- Fat: 15-20g

Cooking Time

- 15 minutes

Turmeric-Spiced French Toast

Ingredients

- 2 slices whole-grain bread
- 1 egg
- 1/4 cup almond milk
- 1/2 teaspoon ground turmeric
- 1/4 teaspoon cinnamon
- 1/2 teaspoon vanilla extract
- 1/2 cup fresh berries (e.g., blueberries, blackberries, and strawberries)

Preparation

- Whisk together egg, almond milk, turmeric, cinnamon, and vanilla extract in a bowl.
- Dip bread slices into the mixture, ensuring they are coated.

- Cook in a heated, non-stick skillet until golden brown on both sides.
- Serve with fresh berries.

Nutritional Value

- Calories: 300-350
- Protein: 10-12g
- Carbohydrates: 35-40g
- Dietary Fiber: 6-8g
- Sugars: 10-15g (from natural sugars in berries)
- Fat: 10-15g

Cooking Time:

- 15 minutes

Bison Sausage Breakfast Burrito

Ingredients

- 1 whole-grain tortilla
- 1/4 cup cooked bison sausage
- 2 scrambled eggs
- 1/4 cup diced tomatoes
- 1/2 teaspoon chopped dill

Preparation

- Warm the tortilla.
- Fill it with cooked bison sausage, scrambled eggs, diced tomatoes, and chopped dill.

Nutritional Value:

- Calories: 350-400
- Protein: 20-25g
- Carbohydrates: 25-30g
- Dietary Fiber: 5-7g
- Fat: 15-20g

Cooking Time:
- 15 minutes

Spinach and Goat Cheese Breakfast Quesadilla

Ingredients
- 1 whole-grain tortilla
- 1/2 cup sautéed spinach
- 1/4 cup crumbled goat cheese
- 1 poached egg

Preparation
- Warm the tortilla.
- Layer with sautéed spinach, crumbled goat cheese, and a poached egg.

Nutritional Value:
- Calories: 350-400
- Protein: 15-20g
- Carbohydrates: 25-30g
- Dietary Fiber: 5-7g
- Fat: 15-20g

Cooking Time:

* 15 minutes

Baked Sweet Potato with Yogurt

Ingredients
* 1 small sweet potato
* 1/2 cup Greek yogurt
* 1 teaspoon honey
* 1 tablespoon chopped walnuts

Preparation
* Bake the sweet potato until tender.
* Slice it open and fill with Greek yogurt.
* Drizzle with honey and sprinkle with chopped walnuts.

Nutritional Value
* Calories: 300-350
* Protein: 15-20g
* Carbohydrates: 35-40g
* Dietary Fiber: 6-8g
* Sugars: 10-15g (from natural sugars in sweet potato and yogurt)
* Fat: 10-15g

Cooking Time
* 45 minutes (mostly for baking the sweet potato)

Papaya Breakfast Boat

Ingredients
- 1 ripe papaya
- 1/2 cup Greek yogurt
- 1 teaspoon honey
- 1 tablespoon toasted coconut flakes

Preparation
- Cut the papaya in half and remove the seeds.
- Fill the papaya halves with Greek yogurt.
- Drizzle with honey and top with toasted coconut flakes

Nutritional Value:
- Calories: 300-350
- Protein: 10-15g
- Carbohydrates: 40-45g
- Dietary Fiber: 6-8g
- Sugars: 25-30g (from natural sugars in papaya and yogurt)
- Fat: 10-15g

Cooking Time:
- 10 minutes

Buckwheat Waffles

Ingredients
- 1 cup buckwheat flour
- 1/2 teaspoon baking powder
- 1 egg

- 1 cup almond milk

Preparation

- Mix buckwheat flour and baking powder.
- In a separate bowl, beat the egg and combine it with almond milk.
- Stir the wet ingredients into the dry to make the waffle batter.
- Cook the waffles in a waffle iron.

Nutritional Value:

- Calories: 300-350
- Protein: 8-10g
- Carbohydrates: 45-50g
- Dietary Fiber: 6-8g
- Sugars: 2-5g
- Fat: 10-15g

Cooking Time:

- 20 minutes

Chia Seed Pudding

Ingredients

- 3 tablespoons chia seeds
- 1 cup almond milk
- 1/2 teaspoon vanilla extract
- 1 teaspoon maple syrup (optional)
- A handful of sliced cherries

Preparation

- In a bowl, mix chia seeds, almond milk, vanilla extract, and maple syrup (if using).
- Stir well to combine.
- Cover and refrigerate the mixture overnight or for at least 4 hours.
- Before serving, give it a good stir.
- Top with sliced cherries.

Nutritional Value:

- Calories: 250-300
- Protein: 5-7g
- Carbohydrates: 20-25g
- Dietary Fiber: 10-12g
- Sugars: 8-10g (from cherries)
- Fat: 10-15g
- Omega-3 Fatty Acids: 4-6g (from chia seeds

Cooking Time:

- 5-10 minutes (preparation time

Smoked Salmon and Spinach Omelet

Ingredients

- 2 eggs
- 1/4 cup diced smoked salmon
- 1/2 cup sautéed spinach
- 1/2 teaspoon chopped dill

Preparation

- Whisk the eggs in a bowl.
- Heat a non-stick skillet over medium heat.
- Add the whisked eggs and allow them to cook undisturbed for a minute or two.
- Add diced smoked salmon and sautéed spinach.
- Sprinkle chopped dill over the omelet.
- Fold the omelet in half and cook until the eggs are set.

Nutritional Value:

- Calories: 250-300
- Protein: 20-25g
- Carbohydrates: 2-5g
- Fat: 15-20g

Cooking Time:

- 10 minutes

Avocado Toast

Ingredients

- 2 slices whole-grain bread
- 1 ripe avocado, mashed
- Red pepper flakes (to taste)
- 2 poached eggs

Preparation

- Toast the slices of whole-grain bread.
- Spread mashed avocado on the toasted bread.
- Sprinkle with red pepper flakes.
- Top each slice with a poached egg.

Nutritional Value:

- Calories: 300-350
- Protein: 15-20g
- Carbohydrates: 25-30g
- Dietary Fiber: 6-8g
- Fat: 15-20g

Cooking Time:

- 15 minutes

CHAPTER 4:LUNCH TIME FAVORITES

NUTRIENT-PACKED LUNCH OPTIONS

Mediterranean Quinoa Salad

Ingredients

- 1 cup cooked quinoa
- 1/2 cup diced cucumber
- 1/2 cup diced tomatoes
- 1/4 cup diced red onions
- 1/4 cup crumbled feta cheese
- 2 tablespoons Kalamata olives
- 2 tablespoons extra virgin olive oil
- 1 tablespoon lemon juice
- 1 teaspoon dried oregano
- Salt and pepper to taste

Preparation

- In a large bowl, combine quinoa, cucumber, tomatoes, red onions, feta cheese, and olives.
- In a small bowl, whisk together olive oil, lemon juice, dried oregano, salt, and pepper.

- Drizzle the dressing over the salad and toss to combine.

Nutritional Value

- Calories: 400-450
- Protein: 10-15g
- Carbohydrates: 40-45g
- Dietary Fiber: 6-8g
- Sugars: 4-6g
- Fat: 20-25g

Cooking Time

- 15 minutes (mostly for quinoa preparation)

Bison and Vegetable Stir-Fry

Ingredients

- 1/2 cup cooked bison meat (sliced)
- 1 cup mixed stir-fry vegetables (broccoli, bell peppers, snap peas)
- 1/4 cup sliced water chestnuts
- 2 tablespoons low-sodium soy sauce
- 1 teaspoon grated fresh ginger
- 1 clove garlic (minced)
- 1 tablespoon sesame oil
- Cooked brown rice (as a base)

Preparation

- In a wok or large skillet, heat sesame oil over medium-high heat.

- Add ginger and garlic, sauté for 1 minute.
- Add bison and stir-fry until cooked.
- Add vegetables and water chestnuts, stir-fry until tender.
- Drizzle with soy sauce and serve over brown rice.

Nutritional Value

- Calories: 400-450
- Protein: 25-30g
- Carbohydrates: 30-35g
- Dietary Fiber: 4-6g
- Sugars: 4-6g
- Fat: 15-20g

Cooking Time

- 20 minutes

Lentil and Vegetable Salad

Ingredients

- 1 cup cooked lentils
- 1/2 cup diced bell peppers (various colors)
- 1/2 cup diced cucumber
- 1/4 cup diced red onions
- 2 tablespoons chopped fresh parsley
- 2 tablespoons lemon juice
- 1 tablespoon extra virgin olive oil

- Salt and pepper to taste

Preparation

- In a large bowl, combine cooked lentils, bell peppers, cucumber, red onions, and fresh parsley.
- In a small bowl, whisk together lemon juice, olive oil, salt, and pepper.
- Drizzle the dressing over the salad and toss to combine

Nutritional Value

- Calories: 350-400
- Protein: 15-20g
- Carbohydrates: 50-55g
- Dietary Fiber: 10-12g
- Sugars: 6-8g
- Fat: 10-15g

Cooking Time

- 15 minutes (mostly for lentil preparation)

Salmon and Quinoa Bowl

Ingredients

- 1 grilled salmon fillet
- 1 cup cooked quinoa
- 1/2 cup steamed asparagus
- 1/4 cup diced avocado
- 1/4 cup diced mango

- 1 tablespoon olive oil
- 1 tablespoon lemon juice
- Fresh dill for garnish

Preparation

- Grill the salmon fillet until cooked through.
- In a bowl, combine cooked quinoa, steamed asparagus, diced avocado, and mango.
- Drizzle with olive oil and lemon juice.
- Top with the grilled salmon and garnish with fresh dill.

Nutritional Value

- Calories: 400-450
- Protein: 25-30g
- Carbohydrates: 40-45g
- Dietary Fiber: 6-8g
- Sugars: 4-6g
- Fat: 15-20g

Cooking Time

- 20 minutes

Turkey and Swiss Cheese Sandwich

Ingredients

- 2 slices whole-grain bread
- 3-4 slices turkey breast
- 2 slices Swiss cheese
- 1/4 cup mixed greens

- 1 tablespoon Dijon mustard
- 1 tablespoon mayonnaise
- 1/2 teaspoon dried basil

Preparation

- Spread Dijon mustard and mayonnaise on one slice of bread.
- Layer turkey, Swiss cheese, mixed greens, and dried basil on the bread.
- Top with the second slice of bread.
- Press gently and slice in half.

Nutritional Value

- Calories: 350-400
- Protein: 20-25g
- Carbohydrates: 25-30g
- Dietary Fiber: 4-6g
- Sugars: 3-5g
- Fat: 15-20g

Cooking Time

- 5 minutes

Avocado and Chicken Wrap

Ingredients

- 1 whole-grain wrap or tortilla
- 1/2 cup cooked chicken breast (shredded)
- 1/4 cup diced tomatoes
- 1/4 cup diced red onions

- 1/4 cup mixed greens
- 1/4 ripe avocado (sliced)
- 1 tablespoon Greek yogurt
- 1 teaspoon lemon juice
- Salt and pepper to taste

Preparation

- In a bowl, combine shredded chicken, diced tomatoes, red onions, and mixed greens.
- In a separate bowl, mix Greek yogurt, lemon juice, salt, and pepper.
- Spread the Greek yogurt mixture on the wrap.
- Add the chicken mixture and avocado slices.
- Roll up the wrap and cut in half.

Nutritional Value

- Calories: 400-450
- Protein: 25-30g
- Carbohydrates: 30-35g
- Dietary Fiber: 6-8g
- Sugars: 4-6g
- Fat: 20-25g

Cooking Time

- 10 minutes (mostly for chicken preparation.

Eggplant and Red Pepper Salad

Ingredients

- 1 small eggplant
- 1 red bell pepper
- 1/4 cup feta cheese (crumbled)
- 2 tablespoons balsamic vinegar
- 1 tablespoon olive oil
- 1/2 teaspoon dried basil
- Salt and pepper to taste

Preparation

- Preheat the oven to 400°F (200°C).
- Slice the eggplant and red bell pepper.
- Place them on a baking sheet, drizzle with olive oil, and sprinkle with dried basil, salt, and pepper.
- Roast in the oven until tender (about 20-25 minutes).
- Let the roasted vegetables cool.
- In a bowl, combine the roasted eggplant and red pepper.
- Drizzle with balsamic vinegar and top with crumbled feta cheese.

Nutritional Value

- Calories: 350-400
- Protein: 10-15g
- Carbohydrates: 25-30g
- Dietary Fiber: 8-10g
- Sugars: 8-10g

- Fat: 15-20g

Cooking Time
- 30-35 minutes

Greek Chicken Salad

Ingredients
- 1 grilled chicken breast (sliced)
- 1 cup mixed greens
- 1/4 cup diced cucumbers
- 1/4 cup diced tomatoes
- 2 tablespoons feta cheese (crumbled)
- 1 tablespoon Kalamata olives
- 2 tablespoons Greek dressing
- Fresh oregano for garnish

Preparation
- Grill the chicken breast until cooked through.
- In a bowl, combine mixed greens, diced cucumbers, tomatoes, crumbled feta cheese, and Kalamata olives.
- Top with grilled chicken slices.
- Drizzle with Greek dressing and garnish with fresh oregano.

Nutritional Value
- Calories: 400-450
- Protein: 25-30g

- Carbohydrates: 10-15g
- Dietary Fiber: 4-6g
- Sugars: 2-4g
- Fat: 20-5g

Cooking Time

- 15 minutes

Quinoa and Black Bean Salad

Ingredients

- 1 cup cooked quinoa
- 1/2 cup canned black beans (drained and rinsed)
- 1/4 cup diced red onions
- 1/4 cup diced bell peppers (various colors)
- 1/4 cup diced tomatoes
- 1/4 cup chopped fresh cilantro
- 2 tablespoons lime juice
- 1 tablespoon olive oil
- 1/2 teaspoon ground cumin
- Salt and pepper to taste

Preparation

- In a bowl, combine cooked quinoa, black beans, red onions, bell peppers, tomatoes, and fresh cilantro.

- In a separate bowl, whisk together lime juice, olive oil, ground cumin, salt, and pepper.
- Drizzle the dressing over the salad and toss to combine.

Nutritional Value
- Calories: 350-400
- Protein: 10-15g
- Carbohydrates: 45-50g
- Dietary Fiber: 8-10g
- Sugars: 4-6g
- Fat: 15-20g

Cooking Time
- 15 minutes (mostly for quinoa preparation

Asian Chicken Lettuce Wraps

Ingredients
- 1 cup cooked chicken breast (diced)
- 1/4 cup diced water chestnuts
- 1/4 cup diced red bell pepper
- 1/4 cup diced green onions
- 2 tablespoons low-sodium soy sauce
- 1 tablespoon hoisin sauce
- 1/2 teaspoon sesame oil
- Lettuce leaves (e.g., iceberg or butter lettuce) for wrapping

Preparation

- In a bowl, combine diced chicken, water chestnuts, red bell pepper, and green onions.
- In a separate bowl, mix soy sauce, hoisin sauce, and sesame oil.
- Drizzle the sauce over the chicken mixture.
- Spoon the chicken mixture into lettuce leaves and wrap them like tacos

Nutritional Value

- Calories: 350-400
- Protein: 25-30g
- Carbohydrates: 15-20g
- Dietary Fiber: 4-6g
- Sugars: 4-6g
- Fat: 15-20g

Cooking Time

- 15 minutes (mostly for chicken preparation

Beef and Vegetable Stir-Fry

Ingredients

- 1/2 cup cooked lean beef (sliced)
- 1 cup mixed stir-fry vegetables (e.g., broccoli, snow peas, carrots)
- 1/4 cup sliced water chestnuts
- 2 tablespoons low-sodium soy sauce

- 1 teaspoon grated fresh ginger
- 1 clove garlic (minced)
- 1 tablespoon sesame oil
- Cooked brown rice (as a base)

Preparation

- In a wok or large skillet, heat sesame oil over medium-high heat.
- Add ginger and garlic, sauté for 1 minute.
- Add sliced beef and stir-fry until heated.
- Add mixed vegetables and water chestnuts, stir-fry until tender.
- Drizzle with soy sauce and serve over brown rice.

Nutritional Value

- Calories: 400-450
- Protein: 25-30g
- Carbohydrates: 30-35g
- Dietary Fiber: 4-6g
- Sugars: 4-6g
- Fat: 20-25g

Cooking Time

- 20 minutes

Pomegranate and Walnut Chicken Salad

Ingredients

- 1 grilled chicken breast (sliced)

- 2 cups mixed greens
- 1/4 cup pomegranate seeds
- 2 tablespoons chopped walnuts
- 2 tablespoons crumbled feta cheese
- 2 tablespoons balsamic vinaigrette

Preparation

- Grill the chicken breast until cooked through.
- In a bowl, combine mixed greens, pomegranate seeds, chopped walnuts, and crumbled feta cheese.
- Top with grilled chicken slices.
- Drizzle with balsamic vinaigrette.

Nutritional Value

- Calories: 400-450
- Protein: 20-25g
- Carbohydrates: 15-20g
- Dietary Fiber: 4-6g
- Sugars: 6-8g
- Fat: 20-25g

Cooking Time

- 15 minutes

Tuna Salad Sandwich

Ingredients

- 2 slices whole-grain bread
- 1 can of tuna in water (drained)
- 2 tablespoons Greek yogurt

- 1/4 cup diced celery
- 1/4 cup diced red onions
- 1/2 teaspoon dried dill
- Lettuce leaves for garnish

Preparation

- In a bowl, mix drained tuna, Greek yogurt, celery, red onions, and dried dill.
- Spread the tuna salad on one slice of bread.
- Top with lettuce leaves and the second slice of bread.
- Slice in half.

Nutritional Value

- Calories: 350-400
- Protein: 20-25g
- Carbohydrates: 20-25g
- Dietary Fiber: 4-6g
- Sugar: 4-6g
- Fat: 15-20g

Cooking Time

- 10 minutes

Shrimp and Avocado Salad

Ingredients

- 1 cup cooked shrimp
- 1/2 ripe avocado (sliced)
- 1/4 cup diced red onions

- 1/4 cup diced cucumber
- 2 cups mixed greens
- 2 tablespoons lemon juice
- 1 tablespoon olive oil
- Fresh cilantro leaves for garnish

Preparation

- In a bowl, combine cooked shrimp, avocado slices, red onions, cucumber, and mixed greens.
- In a small bowl, whisk together lemon juice and olive oil.
- Drizzle the dressing over the salad and garnish with fresh cilantro leaves

Nutritional Value

- Calories: 350-400
- Protein: 20-25g
- Carbohydrates: 15-20g
- Dietary Fiber: 6-8g
- Sugars: 4-6g
- Fat: 20-25g

Cooking Time

- 10 minutes (mostly for shrimp preparation

Mango and Tofu Summer Rolls

Ingredients

- 6 rice paper wrappers
- 1/2 cup diced firm tofu
- 1/2 cup diced mango
- 1/4 cup cooked rice vermicelli noodles
- 1/4 cup fresh basil leaves
- 1/4 cup fresh mint leaves
- 1/4 cup fresh cilantro leaves
- 1/4 cup chopped roasted peanuts
- 2 tablespoons hoisin sauce

Preparation

- Fill a large bowl with warm water.
- Dip a rice paper wrapper in the warm water until it becomes pliable (about 20 seconds).
- Lay the wrapper flat and arrange tofu, mango, rice vermicelli noodles, basil, mint, cilantro, and chopped peanuts on the lower third.
- Fold the sides of the wrapper over the filling, then roll it up tightly.
- Serve with hoisin sauce for dipping.

Nutritional Value

- Calories: 350-400
- Protein: 15-20g

- Carbohydrates: 40-45g
- Dietary Fiber: 6-8g
- Sugar: 10-15g
- Fat: 10-15g

Cooking Time

- 20 minutes

Quinoa and Roasted Vegetable Salad

Ingredients

- 1 cup cooked quinoa
- 1 cup mixed roasted vegetables (bell peppers, zucchini, eggplant)
- 2 tablespoons olive oil
- 1 tablespoon balsamic vinegar
- 2 tablespoons chopped parsley

Preparation

- Toss quinoa and roasted vegetables in olive oil and balsamic vinegar.
- Garnish with chopped parsley.

Nutritional Value

- Calories: 350-400
- Protein: 10-12g
- Carbohydrates: 35-40g
- Dietary Fiber: 5-7g
- Fat: 20-25g

Cooking Time

* 30 minutes

Balsamic Chicken Salad

Ingredients

* 4 ounces grilled chicken breast, sliced
* 2 cups mixed greens (e.g., kale, spinach, arugula)
* 1/4 cup sliced strawberries
* 2 tablespoons crumbled goat cheese
* 1 tablespoon balsamic vinaigrette
* 1 tablespoon chopped walnuts

Preparation

* Arrange mixed greens on a plate.
* Top with sliced chicken, strawberries, and goat cheese.
* Drizzle with balsamic vinaigrette and sprinkle with walnuts.

Nutritional Value

* Calories: 350-400
* Protein: 25-30g
* Carbohydrates: 10-15g
* Dietary Fiber: 2-4g
* Fat: 15-20g

Cooking Time

* 20 minutes

Asian-Inspired Tofu Salad

Ingredients

- 6 oz firm tofu, cubed
- 2 cups mixed greens (e.g., kale, spinach)
- 1/4 cup sliced red bell pepper
- 1/4 cup shredded carrots
- 1 tablespoon sesame seeds
- 2 tablespoons low-sodium soy sauce
- 1 tablespoon rice vinegar

Preparation

- Toss tofu, greens, bell pepper, and carrots in a bowl.
- Drizzle with soy sauce and rice vinegar.
- Sprinkle sesame seeds on top.

Nutritional Value

- Calories: 300-350
- Protein: 15-20g
- Carbohydrates: 15-20g
- Dietary Fiber: 4-6g
- Fat: 15-20g

Cooking Time

- 15 minutes (for tofu preparation

CHAPTER 5:WHOLESOME DINNERS FOR BLOOD TYPE B

MEAT-BASED DISHES

Lemon Herb Grilled Chicken

Ingredients
- 2 boneless, skinless chicken breasts
- 1 lemon, juiced and zested
- 2 cloves garlic, minced
- 1 tablespoon fresh rosemary, chopped
- Salt and pepper to taste

Preparation
- In a bowl, combine lemon juice, lemon zest, garlic, rosemary, salt, and pepper.
- Marinate the chicken in the mixture for 30 minutes.
- Grill the chicken until cooked through, about 15-20 minutes

Nutritional Value
- Calories: 250-300
- Protein: 30-35g
- Carbohydrates: 5-10g
- Fat: 5-10g

Cooking Time
- 30 minutes (including marinating time)

Bison Stir-Fry

Ingredients

- 1/2 lb bison steak, thinly sliced
- 2 cups mixed vegetables (e.g., bell peppers, broccoli, carrots)
- 2 tablespoons low-sodium soy sauce
- 1 tablespoon sesame oil
- 1/2 teaspoon ginger, minced
- 1/2 teaspoon garlic, minced

Preparation

- In a wok or skillet, heat sesame oil over high heat.
- Add bison and stir-fry until browned. Remove and set aside.
- In the same pan, add vegetables, ginger, and garlic. Stir-fry for a few minutes.
- Return bison to the pan, add soy sauce, and stir-fry until heated through.

Nutritional Value

- Calories: 300-350
- Protein: 25-30g
- Carbohydrates: 15-20g
- Dietary Fiber: 4-6g
- Fat: 10-15g

Cooking Time

- 20 minutes

Turkey and Sweet Potato Hash

Ingredients
- 1 lb ground turkey
- 2 sweet potatoes, diced
- 1 onion, diced
- 1 teaspoon paprika
- Salt and pepper to taste

Preparation
- In a skillet, brown ground turkey until cooked through. Remove and set aside.
- In the same pan, sauté sweet potatoes and onions until tender.
- Add cooked turkey back to the pan and season with paprika, salt, and pepper.

Nutritional Value
- Calories: 350-400
- Protein: 25-30g
- Carbohydrates: 30-35g
- Dietary Fiber: 5-7g
- Fat: 10-15g

Cooking Time
- 30 minutes

Lamb and Vegetable Kebabs

Ingredients
- 1 lb lamb cubes
- 2 bell peppers, cut into chunks

- 1 red onion, cut into chunks
- 2 tablespoons olive oil
- 1 teaspoon cumin
- 1/2 teaspoon paprika
- Salt and pepper to taste

Preparation

- In a bowl, combine olive oil, cumin, paprika, salt, and pepper.
- Thread lamb, peppers, and onion onto skewers.
- Brush with the olive oil mixture.
- Grill or broil the kebabs until the lamb is cooked to your desired doneness.

Nutritional Value

- Calories: 300-350
- Protein: 20-25g
- Carbohydrates: 10-15g
- Dietary Fiber: 2-4g
- Fat: 15-20g

Cooking Time

- 15-20 minutes (grilling or broiling time

Lemon and Dill Grilled Shrimp

Ingredients

- 1 lb large shrimp, peeled and deveined
- 2 tablespoons olive oil
- 2 cloves garlic, minced

- Zest and juice of 1 lemon
- 1 tablespoon fresh dill, chopped
- Salt and pepper to taste

Preparation

- In a bowl, mix olive oil, garlic, lemon zest, lemon juice, dill, salt, and pepper.
- Marinate the shrimp in the mixture for 15 minutes.
- Thread the shrimp onto skewers and grill until pink and cooked through, about 5-7 minutes.

Nutritional Value

- Calories: 250-300
- Protein: 30-35g
- Carbohydrates: 5-10g
- Fat: 10-15g

Cooking Time

- 25 minutes (including marinating and grilling time

Pork and Vegetable Stir-Fry

Ingredients

- 1/2 lb pork loin, thinly sliced
- 2 cups mixed vegetables (e.g., broccoli, bell peppers, snap peas)
- 2 tablespoons low-sodium soy sauce
- 1 tablespoon sesame oil

- 1/2 teaspoon ginger, minced
- 1/2 teaspoon garlic, minced

Preparation

- In a wok or skillet, heat sesame oil over high heat.
- Add pork and stir-fry until browned. Remove and set aside.
- In the same pan, add vegetables, ginger, and garlic. Stir-fry for a few minutes.
- Return pork to the pan, add soy sauce, and stir-fry until heated through.

Nutritional Value

- Calories: 350-400
- Protein: 25-30g
- Carbohydrates: 15-20g
- Dietary Fiber: 4-6g
- Fat: 15-20g

Cooking Time

- 20 minutes

VEGETARIAN DISHES

Eggplant and Chickpea Curry

Ingredients

- 1 large eggplant, diced
- 1 can chickpeas, drained and rinsed
- 1 onion, chopped

- 2 cloves garlic, minced
- 1 can diced tomatoes
- 2 tablespoons curry powder
- 1/2 cup coconut milk
- Salt and pepper to taste

Preparation

- In a large pot, sauté onions and garlic until translucent.
- Add eggplant and cook for a few minutes.
- Stir in diced tomatoes, chickpeas, and curry powder.
- Simmer until the eggplant is tender, about 20 minutes.
- Stir in coconut milk and season with salt and pepper.

Nutritional Value

- Calories: 350-400
- Protein: 10-15g
- Carbohydrates: 40-45g
- Dietary Fiber: 10-12g
- Fat: 15-20g

Cooking Time

- 30 minutes

Mushroom and Spinach Stuffed Peppers

Ingredients

- 4 bell peppers
- 2 cups mushrooms, chopped
- 2 cups fresh spinach, chopped
- 1 onion, diced
- 1 cup cooked quinoa
- 1/4 cup grated Parmesan cheese
- Salt and pepper to taste

Preparation

- Preheat the oven to 350°F (175°C).
- Cut the tops off the peppers and remove seeds and membranes.
- In a skillet, sauté mushrooms, spinach, and onions until tender.
- Stir in quinoa, Parmesan cheese, salt, and pepper.
- Stuff each pepper with the mixture and bake for 30-35 minutes.

Nutritional Value

- Calories: 250-300
- Protein: 10-15g
- Carbohydrates: 30-35g
- Dietary Fiber: 5-7g
- Fat: 10-15g

Cooking Time

- 45 minutes (including baking time)

Spinach and Chickpea Stuffed Acorn Squash

Ingredients

- 2 acorn squash, halved and seeds removed
- 2 cups fresh spinach
- 1 can chickpeas, drained and rinsed
- 1/2 cup feta cheese, crumbled
- 1/4 cup chopped fresh parsley
- 2 tablespoons olive oil
- Salt and pepper to taste

Preparation

- Preheat the oven to 400°F (200°C).
- Brush squash halves with olive oil, season with salt and pepper, and roast for 30-40 minutes or until tender.
- In a skillet, sauté spinach until wilted.
- Combine chickpeas, feta cheese, and parsley.
- Stuff the roasted squash halves with the mixture and return to the oven for an additional 10 minutes.

Nutritional Value

- Calories: 350-400
- Protein: 15-20g
- Carbohydrates: 50-55g
- Dietary Fiber: 10-12g
- Fat: 15-20g

Cooking Time

- 50-60 minutes

Vegetarian Red Lentil Curry

Ingredients

- 1 cup red lentils
- 1 onion, chopped
- 2 cloves garlic, minced
- 1 can diced tomatoes
- 1 can coconut milk
- 2 tablespoons curry powder
- Salt and pepper to taste

Preparation

- In a pot, sauté onions and garlic until translucent.
- Stir in red lentils, diced tomatoes, curry powder, salt, and pepper.
- Add coconut milk and simmer for about 20-25 minutes until lentils are tender.

Nutritional Value

- Calories: 300-350
- Protein: 15-20g
- Carbohydrates: 40-45g
- Dietary Fiber: 10-12g
- Fat: 10-15g

Cooking Time

- 30 minutes

Pumpkin and Black Bean Stew

Ingredients

- 2 cups diced pumpkin or butternut squash
- 1 can black beans, drained and rinsed
- 1 onion, diced
- 2 cloves garlic, minced
- 1 can diced tomatoes
- 1 teaspoon chili powder
- Salt and pepper to taste

Preparation

- In a pot, sauté onions and garlic until translucent.
- Add pumpkin, black beans, diced tomatoes, chili powder, salt, and pepper.
- Simmer until the pumpkin is tender, about 20-25 minutes.

Nutritional Value

- Calories: 300-350
- Protein: 10-15g
- Carbohydrates: 60-65g
- Dietary Fiber: 15-18g
- Fat: 5-10g

Cooking Time

- 30 minutes

Vegetarian Thai Green Curry

Ingredients

- 1 cup broccoli florets
- 1 cup sliced bell peppers
- 1 cup sliced zucchini
- 1 can coconut milk
- 2 tablespoons green curry paste
- 1 tablespoon soy sauce
- 1/2 cup tofu, cubed
- Fresh basil leaves (as garnish)

Preparation

- In a pot, combine coconut milk, green curry paste, and soy sauce.
- Add vegetables and tofu. Simmer for 15-20 minutes.
- Garnish with fresh basil leaves before serving.

Nutritional Value

- Calories: 350-400
- Protein: 10-15g
- Carbohydrates: 15-20g
- Dietary Fiber: 4-6g
- Fat: 15-20g

Cooking Time

- 30 minutes

GRAIN-BASED DISHES

Teriyaki Salmon with Brown Rice

Ingredients

- 2 salmon fillets
- 1 cup brown rice, cooked
- 1/4 cup teriyaki sauce
- 1 tablespoon sesame seeds
- Steamed broccoli (as a side)

Preparation

- Grill or broil the salmon fillets and brush with teriyaki sauce.
- Serve over cooked brown rice.
- Sprinkle with sesame seeds and serve with steamed broccoli.

Nutritional Value

- Calories: 350-400
- Protein: 30-35g
- Carbohydrates: 40-45g
- Dietary Fiber: 4-6g
- Fat: 15-20g

Cooking Time

- 20 minutes

Spaghetti Squash with Pesto and Cherry Tomatoes

Ingredients

- 1 spaghetti squash, halved and seeds removed
- 1/4 cup pesto sauce (vegetarian)
- 1 cup cherry tomatoes, halved
- 2 tablespoons grated Parmesan cheese (vegetarian)

Preparation

- Preheat the oven to 375°F (190°C).
- Place squash halves on a baking sheet, cut side down, and roast for 40-45 minutes.
- Scrape the flesh with a fork to create "spaghetti."
- Toss with pesto and cherry tomatoes.
- Top with Parmesan cheese before serving.

Nutritional Value

- Calories: 350-400
- Protein: 10-15g
- Carbohydrates: 35-40g
- Dietary Fiber: 6-8g
- Fat: 15-20g

Cooking Time

- 60 minutes (including roasting time)

Salmon and Asparagus Quinoa Bowl

Ingredients

- 2 salmon fillets
- 1 bunch asparagus, trimmed
- 1 cup cooked quinoa
- 1 tablespoon olive oil
- Lemon zest and juice
- Salt and pepper to taste

Preparation

- Preheat the oven to 400°F (200°C).
- Place salmon and asparagus on a baking sheet.
- Drizzle with olive oil, lemon zest, and lemon juice. Season with salt and pepper.
- Roast for 15-20 minutes.
- Serve over cooked quinoa.

Nutritional Value

- Calories: 350-400
- Protein: 30-35g
- Carbohydrates: 20-25g
- Dietary Fiber: 4-6g
- Fat: 15-20g

Cooking Time

- 25 minutes (including roasting time)

Veggie and Tofu Stir-Fry with Brown Rice

Ingredients

- 1 cup brown rice, cooked
- 6 oz firm tofu, cubed
- 2 cups mixed vegetables (e.g., broccoli, bell peppers, snap peas)
- 2 tablespoons low-sodium soy sauce
- 1 tablespoon sesame oil
- 1/2 teaspoon ginger, minced
- 1/2 teaspoon garlic, minced

Preparation

- In a wok or skillet, heat sesame oil over high heat.
- Add tofu and stir-fry until browned. Remove and set aside.
- In the same pan, add vegetables, ginger, and garlic. Stir-fry for a few minutes.
- Return tofu to the pan, add soy sauce, and stir-fry until heated through.

Nutritional Value

- Calories: 300-350
- Protein: 15-20g
- Carbohydrates: 45-50g
- Dietary Fiber: 6-8g
- Fat: 10-15g

Cooking Time

- 30 minutes

CHAPTER 6:SNACK AND SIDES :HEALTHY OPTIONS FOR ON-THE-GO

HEALTHY SNACK OPTIONS

Hummus and Veggie Sticks

Ingredients
- 1/2 cup hummus
- Carrot sticks, cucumber slices, and bell pepper strips

Preparation
- Wash and cut the vegetables.
- Serve with hummus for dipping.

Nutritional Value
- Calories: 150-200
- Protein: 5-7g
- Carbohydrates: 15-20g
- Dietary Fiber: 5-7g
- Fat: 8-10g

Cooking Time
- 10 minutes

Greek Yogurt and Berries

Ingredients

- 1 cup Greek yogurt
- 1/2 cup mixed berries (e.g., blueberries, strawberries)
- 1 tablespoon honey (optional)

Preparation

- Spoon yogurt into a bowl.
- Top with berries and drizzle with honey, if desired.

Nutritional Value

- Calories: 200-250
- Protein: 15-20g
- Carbohydrates: 20-25g
- Dietary Fiber: 4-6g
- Fat: 8-10g

Cooking Time

- 5 minutes

Almonds and Dried Apricots

Ingredients

- 1/4 cup almonds
- 1/4 cup dried apricots

Preparation

- Simply measure out the almonds and dried apricots

Nutritional Value

- Calories: 200-250
- Protein: 5-7g
- Carbohydrates: 25-30g
- Dietary Fiber: 4-6g
- Fat: 10-15g

Cooking Time

- No cooking required

Cottage Cheese with Pineapple

Ingredients

- 1/2 cup low-fat cottage cheese
- 1/2 cup fresh pineapple chunks

Preparation

- Scoop cottage cheese into a bowl.
- Top with pineapple chunks.

Nutritional Value

- Calories: 150-200
- Protein: 15-20g
- Carbohydrates: 15-20g
- Dietary Fiber: 2-4g
- Fat: 5-7g

Cooking Time

- 5 minutes

Rice Cakes with Avocado

Ingredients

- 2 rice cakes
- 1/2 ripe avocado, mashed
- Red pepper flakes (to taste)

Preparation

- Spread mashed avocado on rice cakes.
- Sprinkle with red pepper flakes.

Nutritional Value

- Calories: 250-300
- Protein: 4-6g
- Carbohydrates: 20-25g
- Dietary Fiber: 5-7g
- Fat: 15-20g

Cooking Time

- 5 minutes

Mixed Nuts Trail Mix

Ingredients

- 1/4 cup mixed nuts (almonds, walnuts, cashews)
- 1/4 cup mixed dried fruits (raisins, apricots, dates)

Preparation

- Combine mixed nuts and dried fruits for a satisfying trail mix

Nutritional Value

- Calories: 200-250
- Protein: 5-7g
- Carbohydrates: 20-25g
- Dietary Fiber: 3-5g
- Fat: 12-15g

Cooking Time

- 2 minutes

SIDE DISHES

Roasted Sweet Potato Wedges

Ingredients

- 2 sweet potatoes, cut into wedges
- 2 tablespoons olive oil
- 1/2 teaspoon paprika
- Salt and pepper to taste

Preparation

- Preheat the oven to 425°F (220°C).
- Toss sweet potato wedges with olive oil, paprika, salt, and pepper.
- Roast for 25-30 minutes, turning once, until tender and golden

Nutritional Value

- Calories: 200-250
- Protein: 2-4g

- Carbohydrates: 30-35g
- Dietary Fiber: 5-7g
- Fat: 8-10g

Cooking Time

- 35 minutes

Cucumber and Tomato Salad

Ingredients

- 1 cucumber, diced
- 2 tomatoes, diced
- 1/4 cup fresh basil, chopped
- 2 tablespoons olive oil
- 1 tablespoon red wine vinegar
- Salt and pepper to taste

Preparation

- Combine cucumber, tomatoes, and fresh basil in a bowl.
- In a separate bowl, whisk together olive oil, red wine vinegar, salt, and pepper.
- Drizzle the dressing over the salad and toss to combine.

Nutritional Value

- Calories: 150-200
- Protein: 2-4g
- Carbohydrates: 10-15g
- Dietary Fiber: 3-5g
- Fat: 8-10g

Cooking Time

- 10 minutes

Stuffed Grape Leaves (Dolmas)

Ingredients

- 1 jar of grape leaves
- 1 cup cooked brown rice
- 1/4 cup pine nuts
- 1/4 cup chopped fresh dill
- 2 tablespoons lemon juice

Preparation

- Rinse and drain grape leaves.
- In a bowl, combine cooked brown rice, pine nuts, fresh dill, and lemon juice.
- Place a spoonful of the mixture on each grape leaf and roll it up

Nutritional Value

- Calories: 200-250
- Protein: 5-7g
- Carbohydrates: 25-30g
- Dietary Fiber: 4-6g
- Fat: 10-15g

Cooking Time

- 30 minutes

Seaweed Salad

Ingredients

- 1 pack seaweed salad mix
- 1 tablespoon sesame oil
- 1 tablespoon rice vinegar

Preparation

- Combine the seaweed salad mix, sesame oil, and rice vinegar.

Nutritional Value

- Calories: 100-150
- Protein: 2-4g
- Carbohydrates: 10-15g
- Dietary Fiber: 4-6g
- Fat: 8-10g

Cooking Time

- 5 minutes

CHAPTER 7:SWEET TREATS DESSERTS THAT ALIGN WITH YOUR BLOOD TYPE

FRUIT-BASED DESSERTS

Mixed Berry Parfait
Ingredients
- 1 cup mixed berries (blueberries, strawberries, raspberries)
- 1 cup Greek yogurt
- 2 tablespoons honey

Preparation
- Layer mixed berries, Greek yogurt, and honey in a glass.

Nutritional Value
- Calories: 150-200
- Protein: 10-15g
- Carbohydrates: 20-25g
- Dietary Fiber: 2-4g
- Fat: 4-6g

Cooking Time
- 5 minutes

Grilled Pineapple with Cinnamon

Ingredients

- 1 pineapple, sliced
- 1 teaspoon ground cinnamon
- 1 tablespoon honey (optional)

Preparation

- Sprinkle pineapple slices with ground cinnamon.
- Grill until caramelized. Drizzle with honey if desired.

Nutritional Value

- Calories: 100-150
- Protein: 1-2g
- Carbohydrates: 25-30g
- Dietary Fiber: 3-5g
- Fat: 0-2g

Cooking Time

- 10 minutes

Mango Sorbet

Ingredients

- 2 ripe mangoes, peeled and diced
- 1/4 cup honey
- Juice of 1 lime

Preparation

- Blend mangoes, honey, and lime juice until smooth.

- Freeze the mixture until it reaches a sorbet-like consistency.

Nutritional Value

- Calories: 150-200
- Protein: 1-2g
- Carbohydrates: 40-45g
- Dietary Fiber: 3-5g
- Fat: 0-2g

Cooking Time

- 15 minutes (plus freezing time)

Baked Apples with Almonds

Ingredients

- 2 apples, cored and halved
- 1/4 cup chopped almonds
- 1 teaspoon ground cinnamon
- 1 tablespoon honey

Preparation

- Fill apple halves with chopped almonds.
- Sprinkle with ground cinnamon and drizzle with honey.
- Bake until apples are tender.

Nutritional Value

- Calories: 200-250
- Protein: 4-6g
- Carbohydrates: 25-30g
- Dietary Fiber: 5-7g
- Fat: 8-10g

Cooking Time

- 25 minutes

FROZEN TREATS

Banana and Almond Butter Ice Cream

Ingredients

- 2 ripe bananas, sliced and frozen
- 2 tablespoons almond butter

Preparation

- Blend frozen banana slices and almond butter until creamy.
- Freeze for a firmer texture.

Nutritional Value

- Calories: 150-200
- Protein: 3-5g
- Carbohydrates: 25-30g
- Dietary Fiber: 3-5g
- Fat: 6-8g

Cooking Time

- 10 minutes (plus freezing time)

Peach and Greek Yogurt Popsicles

Ingredients

- 2 ripe peaches, peeled and diced
- 1 cup Greek yogurt
- 2 tablespoons honey

Preparation

- Blend peaches, Greek yogurt, and honey until smooth.
- Pour into popsicle molds and freeze.

Nutritional Value

- Calories: 150-200
- Protein: 8-10g
- Carbohydrates: 20-25g
- Dietary Fiber: 2-4g
- Fat: 4-6g

Cooking Time

- 15 minutes (plus freezing time)

BAKED GOODIES

Oatmeal and Banana Cookies

Ingredients

- 2 ripe bananas, mashed
- 1 1/2 cups rolled oats
- 1/4 cup raisins
- 1/4 cup chopped walnuts
- 1 teaspoon ground cinnamon

Preparation

- Combine mashed bananas, rolled oats, raisins, chopped walnuts, and ground cinnamon.
- Drop spoonfuls onto a baking sheet and bake until golden.

Nutritional Value

- Calories: 100-150
- Protein: 3-5g
- Carbohydrates: 20-25g
- Dietary Fiber: 3-5g
- Fat: 3-5g

Cooking Time

- 20 minutes

Coconut Date Balls

Ingredients

- 1 cup pitted dates
- 1/2 cup shredded coconut
- 1/4 cup almond meal
- 1/4 cup cocoa powder (unsweetened)

Preparation

- Blend dates, shredded coconut, almond meal, and cocoa powder in a food processor until a sticky dough forms.
- Roll into small balls and refrigerate until firm.

Nutritional Value

- Calories: 150-200
- Protein: 2-4g
- Carbohydrates: 20-25g
- Dietary Fiber: 5-7g
- Fat: 8-10g

Cooking Time

- 15 minutes

Yogurt-Based Delights

Blueberry Yogurt Popsicles

Ingredients

- 1 cup Greek yogurt
- 1 cup blueberries
- 2 tablespoons honey

Preparation

- Blend Greek yogurt, blueberries, and honey until smooth.
- Pour into popsicle molds and freeze.

Nutritional Value

- Calories: 150-200
- Protein: 10-15g
- Carbohydrates: 20-25g
- Dietary Fiber: 2-4g
- Fat: 4-6g

Cooking Time

- 15 minutes (plus freezing time)

Frozen Mango and Coconut Bites

Ingredients

- 1 cup diced mango, frozen
- 1/2 cup shredded coconut
- 1/4 cup coconut milk
- 2 tablespoons honey

Preparation

- Blend frozen mango, shredded coconut, coconut milk, and honey.
- Pour into small molds or ice cube trays and freeze.

Nutritional Value

- Calories: 150-200
- Protein: 1-2g
- Carbohydrates: 20-25g
- Dietary Fiber: 2-4g
- Fat: 6-8g

Cooking Time

- 15 minutes (plus freezing time)

CHOCOLATE AND NUT TREATS

Dark Chocolate-Dipped Strawberries

Ingredients
- 8-10 fresh strawberries
- 1/4 cup dark chocolate (70% cocoa or higher)

Preparation
- Melt dark chocolate in a microwave or over a double boiler.
- Dip strawberries in melted chocolate and let cool.

Nutritional Value
- Calories: 150-200
- Protein: 2-4g
- Carbohydrates: 20-25g
- Dietary Fiber: 3-5g
- Fat: 6-8g

Cooking Time
- 10 minutes

Chocolate and Almond Clusters

Ingredients

- 1/2 cup dark chocolate chips (70% cocoa or higher)
- 1/2 cup almonds, chopped

Preparation

- Melt dark chocolate chips and mix with chopped almonds.
- Drop spoonfuls onto a parchment paper-lined tray and let cool.

Nutritional Value

- Calories: 150-200
- Protein: 4-6g
- Carbohydrates: 15-20g
- Dietary Fiber: 3-5g
- Fat: 8-10g

Cooking Time

- 15 minutes (plus cooling time)

CONCLUSION

This Blood Type B Diet Cookbook offers a comprehensive guide to embracing a diet tailored to your unique blood type, with a focus on enhancing your health and well-being. The recipes, meal plans, and nutritional insights provided are designed to help you make informed dietary choices that align with the principles of the Blood Type B diet.

Throughout this cookbook, you have explored the scientific foundations, the role of lectins, and the intricate relationship between blood type and digestion. You have delved into the specific foods that are recommended and those to avoid, allowing you to curate a personalized eating plan. From breakfast to dinner and snacks to desserts, these recipes offer a wide range of delicious options that cater to your dietary needs while promoting balanced nutrition.

It's important to remember that adopting and adapting to the Blood Type B diet is not just about what you eat—it's a lifestyle choice that can lead to improved health and vitality. By understanding your unique traits and characteristics associated with Blood Type B, you can harness the power of food as medicine. The health benefits of this diet, such as better digestion, nutrient absorption, and overall well-being, can be truly transformative.

As you embark on this journey, remember that every meal is an opportunity to nourish your body and soul. The Blood Type B diet empowers you to make conscious choices that will not only enhance your health but also enrich your life. It's a reminder that food can indeed be a powerful form of preventative medicine.

So, dear reader, I encourage you to embrace this dietary approach with an open heart and a curious palate. Let this cookbook be your guide as you embark on a journey towards a healthier, more vibrant you. The journey may have its challenges, but the rewards are boundless—improved digestion, balanced energy levels, and a sense of well-being that will enrich every aspect of your life.

Here's to your health, happiness, and a future filled with delicious meals that nourish your body and soul. May the Blood Type B diet become your key to unlocking your full potential and achieving the vibrant health you deserve.

Cheers to your transformative journey ahead!

Jade E.Corry